C000051299

30 Simple Habits for Losing Belly Fat

An easier way to strengthen your body, upgrade your health, improve your appearance and enjoy a better life.

Armin Bergmann

No part of this book or any of its contents may be reproduced, copied, modified or adapted, without the prior written consent of the author, unless otherwise indicated for stand-alone materials.

This book is intended for informational purposes, but should not be considered a substitute for the professional advice of a doctor who is well acquainted with your specific medical needs. Be certain to consult your personal physician before attempting any dietary or weight-loss program.

Introduction

Are you trying to lose belly fat, but it feels like your body and your mind aren't cooperating with your efforts to do so? Could you use a little motivation and some practical advice to help you get the process kickstarted?

Losing weight is the aspiration of just about every adult in our culture. As we age, our metabolism slows down and our stress level increases. Each year, we put on a few more pounds and we gradually become less happy with how we look in the mirror or how we appear in pictures. We tell ourselves that we're going to make changes and finally lose some of the fat that has started to accumulate around our mid-section, but that never seems to happen.

Losing belly fat may seem difficult, but it's honestly not as complicated as we often think it is. The truth is that if we learn to alter some of our daily habits in relatively simple ways, we can lose belly fat and become healthier faster than we may realize.

In this concise book, I'll show you 30 simple habits that are utilized all the time by people of all ages who desire to maintain a healthy weight and a healthy appearance. The habits in this book aren't rocket science, and they don't require you to buy cart loads of weird foods or do a crazy amount of exercise. All I'm suggesting is that if you gradually implement these super simple habits into your daily routine, you'll quickly be pleased with the results. The more habits you consistently implement, the more belly fat you'll gradually lose, the healthier you'll feel and the better you'll look.

This book is for information and motivation purposes only. While it's content is helpful, it is not a substitute for the specific counsel of a doctor who is fully acquainted with your specific health needs. This book is not intended as a substitute for the medical advice of your physician. The reader should regularly consult a physician in matters relating to his/her health and particularly with respect to any symptoms that may require diagnosis or medical attention.

That being said, I wish you all the best on your journey and I hope the content of this book provides the perfect spark of motivation that you need as you march down this road toward better health.

--

1. Don't fill your head with negative self-talk.

Before we talk about some of the physical habits that we can implement in our efforts to lose belly fat, we need to address something in the mental or thought realm that for most people is the **biggest obstacle** they need to overcome in order to be successful in their effort to lose weight.

Of all the voices that we hear every day, our own voice tends to be the one we listen to the most. Sometimes we hear ourselves speaking out loud, but more often than not, our voice speaks messages like a recording on repeat in our minds. We tell ourselves all kinds of things. We're always talking to ourselves in some fashion or another.

"I like this!"

"This makes me happy!"

"I deserve a break."

"Is this day going to drag on forever?"

"This isn't something that I'm good at."

"I'll never get this right."

In the midst of our "self-talk", we can fill our heads with all kinds of information and biases and if we've been struggling to lose belly fat for a long time without success, one of the biggest issues that might be getting in our way is our constant "negative self-talk." We tell ourselves that we're never going to succeed at this and then we fulfill that prophecy by living like a failure, even though that doesn't need to be true.

If other people can lose belly fat, you can too. You're made from the same stuff they're made from. Stop telling yourself that you can't succeed because the more you fill your mind with that notion, the more you'll start living like you've already failed.

One of the habits that is consistently implemented by those who succeed at losing their belly fat is the practice of noticing their negative self-talk and replacing it with a more optimistic assessment. This may be the largest hurdle you need to get through if you've been struggling to lose weight and that's why we're addressing it first. This may be the biggest mountain you need to climb if you're going to maintain the motivation you need to implement the other habits in our list.

If other people can lose belly fat, you can too. Don't forget it. Keep repeating it to yourself. Set yourself up for success by replacing your negative self-talk with a healthy word of encouragement.

2. Stop comparing yourself to others.

We're all similar and we're all made up of the same stuff, but we're not all exactly the same. We all have unique personalities and live and work in unique contexts. We all have unique backgrounds and have experienced unique things on our journey.

It's true that if others can lose belly fat, we can too, but we need to remember that we're all at different places in our journey. That being the case, we need to free ourselves from comparing ourselves to others.

We all know people that seem beautiful in every way and because we tend to get down on ourselves, it's easy to over-analyze ourselves. We stare at our faces in the mirror and wish our noses, chins, ears, eyes and hair looked differently. We look at our profiles and we aren't happy about the pudge that hangs over our belt lines. Then we look at others that are at a different place in their journey and we tell ourselves, "I wish I could look like them," or,

"I wish my body fat was as low as theirs."

Our constant habit of making comparisons is another discourager that we need to identify and avoid. We're all intentionally different and part of maturing as a person is coming to accept those God-ordained differences.

For the sake of our long-term success, let's leave the comparison trap. You're not exactly like the people you idolize and they're not exactly like you and that's perfectly fine. Accept that, embrace that and move on with your personal goals.

3. Set reasonable goals.

While it would be nice to lose 50 lbs. in a week or two, that's not how our bodies function. One of the bad habits we often engage in is the tendency to establish unreasonable goals for ourselves in our weight loss journey. We start the week by saying, "OK, this week I'm going to lose 7 lbs." Then at the end of the week we step on the scale and get disappointed because we only lost 3 lbs.

The truth is that during the first few weeks of implementing the habits of this book, it's common to lose 5 or more lbs. in a week. Some people lose even more. But that's largely based on how much weight you have to lose as well as genetic and environmental factors that are unique to each individual person. In coming weeks, it's more common to lose 1-2 lbs. per week.

But think about that for a second. If I told you that in a few weeks you might weigh 4-8 lbs. less than you do now, do you think you'd be happy about that?　What if I told you that the next time you visit with your extended family, you'll be down 20 lbs.?　How would that sound?

The point I'm making is that it's important to set reasonable goals.　Obviously we all have the long-term goal in mind of having the perfect physique, but in the meantime, let's do ourselves the favor of setting some short-term goals that are achievable and worth celebrating.

If you lose one pound this week, are you going to celebrate that as a victory or get upset that you didn't lose 10 lbs.?　If you lose 8 lbs. this month, are you going to celebrate that even if nobody notices your weight loss?　If your favorite jeans start to fit better, are you going to celebrate that or are you going to get upset because you aren't down three sizes yet?

Get in the habit of setting reasonable goals and then celebrating when you reach them.　Be patient with yourself and show yourself an ample amount of grace.　This is a marathon, not a sprint.

4. Eat only if you're really hungry.

One of the bad habits that we can easily adopt over the course of our lives is eating for just about every reason other than genuine hunger. When we're happy, we eat. When we're feeling a little sad or discouraged, we eat. When we're celebrating, we eat. When we're mourning, we eat. When we're being social, we eat. When we're all alone, we eat. No wonder why we struggle with our mid-sections. We're never giving our stomach a break.

Some people (possibly you), snack constantly. They've got candy on their desk, in their purse and in their car. They eat three meals a day, then a fourth around 10:00 PM and fill in all the empty spaces between meals with sugary or salty snacks and drinks. Have you ever wondered what it would look like to pile up everything you've eaten over the course of a day into one pile on the center of your kitchen table? Every meal. Every snack. Every drink. For some of us, that would be a large pile.

One of the habits that is consistently implemented by those who lose belly fat is that they learn to eat only when they're hungry. And we're talking about physical hunger, not emotional hunger. Our emotions can trick our brains into believing that we need food even when we don't. This happens because we've learned to use food as a mood-altering substance - like a drug.

If you're looking to reach your long-term goals, it's time to engage in the habit of only eating when your body needs food for its natural functions and health. It's time to get out of the habit of feeding our emotions.

5. Get enough sleep.

The body has a natural rhythm that we would do well to pay attention to. We have been designed to consume a certain amount of calories during the day and then rest at night. If we aren't getting the kind of sleep we need, we tend to throw off this rhythm and put ourselves in a position where our bodies are going to function in more of a deprivation mode.

Sleep is an important part of health that shouldn't be ignored. When we develop the habit of getting ample sleep (6.5 - 8 hours / night), we have more energy for the tasks of the day. Likewise, our stress levels are lessened and our emotional resistance to over-eating is strengthened.

When we get enough sleep, our motivation level tends to remain higher as well. But our culture doesn't value sleep as it ought to. We value "burning the midnight oil" instead of enjoying adequate rest and we pride ourselves on telling others that we don't require as much sleep as they do.

But if you ask a majority of those who have consistently maintained a healthy weight for long periods of time, you will notice a pattern in their answers. Most people who are successful with their weight loss and maintenance goals are also getting enough sleep each evening. This is an important habit that we cannot overlook.

6. Eat this kind of breakfast.

Most people agree that breakfast is a pretty important meal. Of all the meals in the day, it's the meal when you can let yourself indulge a little. It can provide a nice energy boost, increase morning productivity and help you resist the urge to over-indulge at lunch time.

All that being said, it may be that you're in the habit of eating the wrong things for breakfast. If your breakfast typically consists of things like cereals (even some of the so-called "healthy" ones), donuts, toast, muffins, jelly, biscuits and other starchy or sugary foods, you're actually in the habit of increasing your belly fat, not reducing it.

Instead of indulging in these sugary, carby and starchy foods, consider eating a breakfast that incorporates more proteins, nuts, fruits and vegetables. This is actually a pattern of eating that we would do well to utilize throughout the day. Omelets, sliced fruit and smoothies are great options to get the day started. Even breakfast meats like bacon, sausage and ham can help contribute to the loss of belly fat when enjoyed in moderation.

The reason we struggle to make eating a "smart" breakfast a daily habit is because it takes more planning than eating cereals, toasts, muffins and donuts. But filling up on proteins, nuts, fruits and veggies keeps us feeling full longer and can help us control our appetite well into the day.

7. Stop eating at least three hours before you go to sleep.

One of the more difficult habits for many people to implement is the concept of "shutting down the kitchen" after dinner. After a long day of work and errands, it's nice to sit down for some TV and unwind after dinner. Usually, after we've had a chance to rest for a couple hours, we start developing an urge for something to munch on, but it's best to get in the habit of resisting that urge so we don't rob ourselves of an evening "fast."

During the night as we rest, our metabolism slows down and our body utilizes the calories and nutrients we consumed during the day for energy. This time of rest is a great time to burn a little fat, provided that our body doesn't need to spend these hours processing and digesting food that was consumed just before sleep.

When we consume unneeded calories just before bed, instead of burning fat while we sleep, we're actually storing up additional fat, most visibly around our mid-section. And to make matters worse, our bodies typically feel hungrier in the morning if we ate just before sleep than they do if we stopped eating after dinner. This may then result in us eating even more unnecessary calories during breakfast.

All that being said, it's best to get in the habit of calling it quits on eating at least three hours before going to sleep.

8. Reduce or eliminate your alcohol intake.

Half the people that read this book will probably skip right over this habit because it isn't what they want to hear, but for those of you who are serious about seeing some noticeable changes in the amount of belly fat you carry around, I would strongly consider this suggestion.

For many people, alcohol is a crutch that they utilize to help dull the pain of their emotional anxieties and life stresses. Some become quite dependent on its presence in their lives and the thought of giving it up is something that they would seriously struggle to consider.

Yet alcohol is a major contributor to the problem of excess belly fat. After it is ingested, the body turns it into sugar, just as it does with breads and grains. If it is being consumed where there is a lack of caloric deficit, it is then stored as fat which most often most visibly accumulates around the waist.

If you're trying to banish your belly, alcohol is not your friend. That's why those who are serious about losing belly fat develop the habit of reducing its consumption or completely eliminating it from their diet altogether.

9. Find a buddy to exercise with and keep each other accountable.

Let's just admit it... developing a long-term pattern of regular exercise is difficult. Even if the exercise we're doing is something routine and enjoyable, it's very easy to talk ourselves out of it more often than we talk ourselves into it.

One habit that is commonly employed by those who have the most success losing weight is finding a buddy that shares your goals. This is helpful on quite a few levels.

A buddy can...

>...help you feel motivated on the days when you're really struggling

>...cheer you on when you meet one of your short-term goals

>...hold you accountable to your

27

long-term goals

...lend you their will-power when yours feels depleted

...join you when you're walking or getting other forms of exercise

...make your exercise times more conversational which help make them go by quicker

...be a listening ear when you need to speak with someone who understands

Finding a buddy to join you isn't very difficult. Most of us know people in our family or work contexts that are probably also looking for an exercise buddy. Sometimes it's just a matter of letting people know that you're looking for a buddy to join you on the journey. You'll probably be surprised to discover several people that might be interested in partnering with you.

The odds of your long-term success in this

effort increase ten-fold if you ask a buddy to join you.

10. Eat slowly.

Being hungry is not a comfortable feeling. When I'm hungry, I usually want the discomfort of hunger to end as quickly as possible. My natural inclination is to eat as much food as I possibly can with the thought that the hunger will go away faster if I eat quicker. But that's not what really happens.

From the moment we begin eating, it takes a little while, often about 20 minutes or so, for our brains to realize we're full. That's why we typically feel terrible just a little while after eating at a buffet. We keep eating and eating without realizing that we're already full.

But when we develop the habit of eating slower, we give the receptors in our brain enough time to give us the "full signal" before we've consumed more calories than we truly need. Slowing down to eat helps us to avoid the error of devouring more than we truly need to eat. It also allows us to enjoy the taste of our food longer which can be especially helpful if we're trying to eat smaller portions.

11. Use a smaller plate to help control portions.

One of the easiest habits in our list to implement is the practice of using a smaller plate. Plates come in all sizes and many of us feel that it's necessary to fill our plate when dining, regardless of its size. That means that most often, if we're using a larger plate, we'll end up eating a larger portion. And eating larger portions means we're going to ingest more calories than we truly need which in turn produces more adipose tissue around our belly.

A simple solution to help address this is to use a smaller plate. When we use a smaller plate, we're still very likely to fill up the available space on that plate when we're portioning out food to ourselves. But because the plate is smaller, we're effectively consuming less while tricking our brains into thinking that we're actually eating a large portion.

12. Fill your sandwiches with vegetables.

Sandwiches are a lunchtime staple. They're a convenient food to eat because they're easy to make and don't require silverware, or a plate for that matter. Many people eat sandwiches at lunchtime at least six out of seven days of the week.

One habit that many people who have successfully reduced their belly fat tend to implement is to fill their sandwiches with vegetables. This isn't to say that they skip on the meats or cheeses or even the mayonnaise. Why is it such a good idea to pack a sandwich full of veggies?

The most obvious benefit is the nutritional and fiber-rich content of the vegetables and that's certainly good to add to your diet. But a less obvious benefit is the fact that packing your sandwich with veggies will help you feel satiated faster and if you're feeling full, you'll be less likely to eat a bag of chips, crackers or cookies with your sandwich to make up for the skimpy content that you put between the slices of bread.

Eating a diet rich in vegetables helps you lose belly fat because vegetables aren't calorie dense. They are also packed with vitamins and fiber which helps with digestion. They're worth filling up on because they're helping your body reach your ultimate goal and they help influence you to avoid filling up on empty calories from snack foods.

13. Weigh yourself daily at first, then weekly afterward.

When you first start implementing the habits in our list, you're likely to notice some quick results. The first few weeks of making changes like this can produce some encouraging numbers on the scale. When you see those numbers start to change, you should let yourself be happy about that and you should let yourself take a peek at the scale each morning because you're likely to see noticeable changes in short periods of time.

Some of the initial weight you'll lose will be water weight which tends to come off quicker than pure fat. Once that excess water is out of your system, the numbers on the scale will begin to change slower. That's perfectly fine. Don't let that discourage you.

Once you move into that stage, stop weighing yourself every day. You'll be used to the numbers moving quicker and it can become discouraging once the process appears to be slowing down. If you keep weighing yourself everyday at this stage, it can become easy to start viewing each day as "good" or "bad" based on whatever that scale is telling you. You don't want to do that to yourself because it will kill your motivation.

A better habit at this stage is to weigh yourself weekly or even bi-weekly (if you can resist). You'll feel better about your progress as you stretch out the time between weigh-ins and will in turn be more likely to continue to implement other habits that help you reach your ultimate goal.

14. Drink mostly water and drink plenty of it.

This habit might seem a little counter-intuitive at first, but let me assure you, it's great habit to implement.

In our culture, many people spend most of their day consuming high-calorie, heavily sweetened beverages. When they have coffee or tea, they add sugar. When they aren't drinking something hot, they're drinking a soda or some kind of juice. Over the course of the day, it's easy to drink an extra 500-800 calories just from the beverage choices we're making. Just imagine what it would do to your waist-line if you dropped 3500-5600 calories from your diet each week. Some people would lose one to two pounds from that change alone.

Keeping our bodies hydrated with water is helpful in many ways. Water helps aid in digesting what we've consumed. It makes us feel full and results in us eating less. It's calorie free so it doesn't result in added fat around our mid-section. It flushes toxins out of our system. It flushes excess sodium out of our system as well which is important because excess sodium can cause us to retain water weight.

On the surface, it would seem that drinking a healthy amount of water throughout the day would actually add to our weight, but it doesn't because it helps keep us full and it flushes some of the excesses out of our system which results in an overall decrease, not an increase in weight.

15. Change what you snack on.

Do you have a sweet-tooth or do you prefer salty snacks? In most kitchens in our culture, you can find cabinets and pantries that are filled with all kinds of goodies (sometimes even taking up more space than canned or jarred foods). We enjoy chips, cookies, candies and we really love our ice cream. These are our go-to foods during those slow moments between meals or later in the evening when we're relaxing. In some cases, these are the biggest culprits in our weight gain. We still seem to think we can eat like we did when we were teenagers, but the truth is our bodies aren't burning calories like they did back then nor are we getting as much physical activity as we did when we were at that stage of life.

So what are we supposed to do when we're hungry, but it isn't a meal time? In those moments, we really have two options if we actually want to succeed in our efforts to reduce body fat. We can either tough it out and live with the hunger or we can allow ourself to enjoy snacks that aren't working against us. Both options are perfectly acceptable.

This habit can be quite difficult for many people, but it's one of the biggest difference-makers in producing lasting change. If you decide not to implement this habit, you'll set yourself back and you won't see the results you want. If you purpose to follow through with this habit, you'll be glad you did.

Some of the things that I like to snack on if I'm really hungry are almonds (in moderation), celery, sliced fruit, some slices of pepperoni and cheese, etc. Basically, what I'm trying to avoid is snacking on sugary, starchy, high-carbohydrate foods. Most of the time, to be honest, I try not to snack at all between meals, but if you're going to snack on something, do yourself the favor and avoid the chips, cake and candy.

16. Spend less time in front of your TV/Computer/Phone.

What do you do at the end of the day? If you're like most people, you probably sit down in front of your TV, computer or mobile device and stare at it while it entertains you. That's perfectly fine to do, provided that it isn't the only thing you do. For some people, this is a 4 to 5 hour evening ritual and they wonder why they keep gaining weight. They sit at a desk all day, snacking, eating high-calorie foods and drinks then come home, eat dinner and sit in front of a TV all evening snacking some more until they fall asleep. The most physical activity they get is when they walk to their car after work or walk to the mailbox to check their mail.

A better habit is to spend a little less time sitting sedentary during the evenings. There are other things that we can incorporate into that time period if we really wanted to, even if we're trying to take care of children.

We can take on a small project around the house, play a little more with the kids, take the dog for a walk or spend some time doing some light cardio exercise. It doesn't have to be complicated, but incorporating a little more physical movement during the evening instead of additional sedentary time can be a great habit that contributes in meaningful ways to our overall goals.

17. Eat fewer processed foods.

If you're struggling with your weight and you're unhappy with the appearance of your mid-section, it's probably a good idea for you to have an honest conversation with yourself about what you're eating. While exercise is important and valuable, the truth is that most weight loss goals can be met through proper nutrition alone.

If you're struggling to lose weight, it may have something to do with the amount of processed foods you're eating. Even though we all enjoy cookies, snack cakes and other packaged foods and snacks, the truth is that the best food we can consume is the food that's closest to its natural state. If we're primarily eating foods that are made from ingredients that we cannot correctly pronounce, we're not doing ourselves any favors in our efforts to lose belly fat.

Processed foods are notorious for being filled with added oils, sugar and sodium. They're also packed with all kinds of weird coloring agents, food preservatives and additives. These foods are usually calorie-heavy and more difficult for our bodies to digest. Eating a diet that primarily consists of processed foods is a recipe for weight gain.

A better habit to implement is to eat foods that are closest to their natural state. Chicken, green beans, carrots, apples, bananas, etc. Our bodies appreciate the nutrition they receive from this kind of diet and will likewise reward our efforts with a slimmer waist-line.

18. Regularly remind yourself of your reasons for losing weight.

We're more than half way through this book which tells me that this would be a good time to mention a habit that is often incorporated by those who succeed in their efforts to reduce belly fat. Those who succeed tend to regularly remind themselves of their reasons for losing weight. They write their reasons down and stare at their lists. They share their reasons with others who are likely to encourage (not discourage) them in their efforts.

Why do you want to reduce your belly fat? If it's because you want to look better, then remind yourself of that regularly. If it's because you want to improve your health, then remind yourself of that. If it's because you're concerned about developing Type-2 diabetes or some other medical concern, then remind yourself of that. If it's to make your spouse, children or parents proud of you, then remind yourself of that.

We all need to find a source of motivation and we ought to keep that source of motivation fresh in our minds so we don't forget why we embarked on this journey to begin with. This is an important habit to implement because it directly relates to our long-term stamina and willingness to complete this journey.

19. Don't eat at restaurants as much.

For many of us, eating out is one of our favorite activities. We enjoy the atmosphere, the opportunity to get out and do something different, the socialization and the great tasting food options. It was recently reported that on average, 9% of the average household budget is spent eating out at restaurants. Depending on your income, that works out to be the cost of a pretty decent home renovation project or a low-mileage used car.

Watching what we eat when we're at restaurants isn't always as easy as we would like it to be. Some restaurants have certainly improved the information that they make available to customers about the ingredients they use and the nutritional content of their meals, but even still, that information isn't always readily available or accessible in easy ways. Most often, we really have no idea what we're really eating at restaurants.

Some restaurants go pretty heavy on added

ingredients like salt, sugar and cooking oils. Their goal isn't to worry about your waist-line. They just want you to really enjoy the taste of what you're eating so you'll keep coming back time and again. And their system is obviously working because many of us are eating at restaurants more times in a week than we care to admit.

If you're serious about shedding excess belly fat, it's time to develop the habit of eating at restaurants a little less. I realize that they're one of our favorite guilty pleasures, but our long-term goals need to start taking precedence over the fickle inclinations of our taste buds.

20. Give yourself an occasional fiber boost.

If you've spent any time watching TV commercials, you've probably heard many different food companies promoting the fact that their foods are "fiber-rich". In some cases it's true. In other cases, these claims are exaggerated, but the truth is that eating fiber-rich foods can be a big help when you're trying to slim down your waist-line.

The unpleasant truth of the matter is that some of the bloating that contributes to our expanding mid-section isn't necessary related to excess fat alone. In many cases, it has much to do with excess waste that we're carrying around within our digestive systems. The thought of that is pretty gross, but it's true. Giving yourself a fiber boost can help correct that problem.

Fiber benefits our bodies in many ways and every time you do something that benefits the overall health of your body, you're also going to directly or indirectly benefit the appearance of your mid-section.

Some of the helpful benefits of fiber are...

> ...It helps to normalizes bowel movements and expel excess waste from our system.

> ...It helps maintain bowel health.

> ...It lowers cholesterol levels.

> ...It is believed to also help prevent colorectal cancer (although studies on this subject are still mixed).

> ...It helps control blood sugar levels.

> ...It aids in losing weight and thereby helps reduce belly fat

Some great sources of fiber that are worth getting in the habit of adding to our diets are; oats, peas, beans, apples, citrus fruits, carrots, barley, whole-wheat flour, wheat bran, nuts, beans and vegetables, such as cauliflower, green beans and potatoes.

Note: Please go light on the grains and starches. They are fine in moderation, but it's more productive to get the bulk of our fiber from fruits and vegetables when we're trying to lose weight.

21. Take long and short walks.

One of the biggest reasons people fail to consistently implement healthy lifestyle habits related to their diet and exercise is because they're choosing options that are too drastic for them and won't be consistently utilized. This is particularly true when it comes to physical exercise.

Every year, gym memberships spike in January as people become serious about losing weight. For several weeks, these new gym members stretch and strain themselves. They spend hours on elliptical machines, treadmills and other workout devices. They leave covered in sweat and exhausted. Then, before they know it, they stop going to the gym because they lose motivation.

One of my favorite habits on our list is this one - the habit of taking walks. Walking is beneficial on so many levels. It gives us the opportunity to enjoy the outdoors. It gets our bodies moving. It can be conversational when enjoyed with a friend and it burns calories and tones muscle.

Some days, you'll have the time and desire to take a long walk. If so, then go for it. Other days, you'll only have time to sneak in a quick walk. That's fine too. It's good to do both. Even a quick 15-minute walk will do more to reduce belly fat than an extra 15 minutes on the couch. And if the weather is favorable, you probably won't become overly sweaty and smelly.

On days when the weather isn't cooperative, taking a walk around an indoor shopping center or a brief walk on a treadmill can do the trick.

22. Don't be afraid to lift a little.

As we mentioned in the previous section, engaging in exercise can be one of the biggest obstacles that gets in the way of people experiencing weight loss success. The good news is that most people can lose weight just fine if they watch what they eat, but certain forms of exercise can provide a nice boost in surprising ways.

You might be surprised by the benefits you'll experience around the mid-section when you start lifting a little weight. And I'm not talking about lifting heavy weights every day of the week. I'm talking about getting in the habit of using a few dumbbells that carry just enough weight that curling them 15 times per each arm is the max you can do at a time without a brief rest.

An objection I often hear to this suggestion relates to the fear of "bulking up." People, particularly women, are afraid that lifting a little weight will make them bulky, but that's not the case at all. Lifting will tone and strengthen the muscles in your back, neck, arms and midsection. Stronger muscles can also help improve posture and thereby visibly reduce the size of our mid-section.

Muscles also do a great job of burning calories for us, and therefore aid us in reducing our storage of excess fat.

23. Avoid diet products and chemical sweeteners.

A common approach to weight loss that is utilized by many people is the consumption of "diet" food products and chemical sweeteners. The marketing divisions of many food companies have done an excellent job in convincing the general public that if we eat the special foods they have developed in their laboratories, our bodies will quickly slim down and our belly fat will be eliminated. This just is not true.

It's best to get in the habit of avoiding diet products and chemical sweeteners all together because these things are just as bad for us, and possibly worse, than other processed foods.

Some scientists are coming to believe that chemical sweeteners in particular can have damaging neurological effects. In addition to that, they don't actually succeed at doing what they claim to do - namely, reduce fat. It has been shown that the body tends to treat chemical sweeteners in some ways as if they were added refined sugar and then store additional fat accordingly.

Psychologically speaking, because we're convinced that we're eating less calories when we ingest diet products, we tend to over-indulge in them and in many cases consume more than we would have if our minds hadn't been tricked into thinking that we were doing something that was better for our body.

Developing the habit of avoiding diet products and chemical sweeteners can be a big help when you're trying to lose excess weight (even though the food processing companies will probably never admit this).

24. Eat as little sugar as possible.

Refined sugar is in many of the processed foods and snacks that we eat. If you look at nutrition labels, you will discover many words that end with "ose". This is code for added sugar, but added sugar goes by quite a few names when it's used in processed food. Here's a few...

*Agave Nectar
*Barley Malt Syrup
*Beet Sugar
*Brown Rice Syrup
*Brown Sugar
*Cane Crystals
*Cane Sugar
*Coconut Sugar, or Coconut Palm Sugar
*Corn sweetener
*Corn syrup, or corn syrup solids
*Dehydrated Cane Juice
*Dextrin
*Dextrose
*Evaporated Cane Juice

*Fructose
*Fruit juice concentrate
*Glucose
*High-fructose corn syrup
*Honey
*Invert sugar
*Lactose
*Maltodextrin
*Malt syrup
*Maltose
*Maple syrup
*Molasses
*Palm Sugar
*Raw sugar
*Rice Syrup
*Saccharose
*Sorghum or sorghum syrup
*Sucrose
*Syrup
*Treacle
*Xylose

Natural sugars that are consumed when eating fruit are usually no big deal. If they aren't eaten in excess, they won't contribute to weight gain or belly fat and the added fiber in the fruit will help with digestion.

Processed foods, on the other hand, tend to be filled with large amounts of added sugar. Eating all of this excess sugar is a bad habit to develop when trying to reduce belly fat. A better habit is to try to avoid it as much as is reasonably possible. As was mentioned earlier, one of the most effective ways to do this is to primarily eat unprocessed foods in their natural state.

Added sugar means added calories and excess calories result in excess fat. For most people, our excess fat gets stored around our mid-section and hips. Reducing the amount of processed sugar in our diet is a habit that helps us reduce belly fat while improving our overall nutritional health.

25. Reduce carbs, grains and starches.

I was once asked by a friend, "What does a farmer feed a pig if he wants to fatten him up?" It was a good question and I pondered it for a moment. Initially, we might think that if a farmer wanted to make a pig fatter, he would feed it something fatty, but that's not the case at all. If a farmer wants to fatten a pig, he doesn't feed it meats and cheeses, he feeds it excess grain and carbohydrates. Our bodies respond is a similar way.

For this reason, it's best to get in the habit of reducing the carbohydrates, grains and starches we choose to eat.

According to Barry Groves at DiabetesHealth.com,

> *"Carbs and carbs alone, not fat, increase body weight..... A short time after a carb-rich meal, the glucose in your bloodstream rises rapidly, and your pancreas*

produces a large amount of insulin to take the excess glucose out.

Just as eating fat doesn't raise blood glucose, it doesn't raise insulin levels either. This is important because insulin is the hormone responsible for body fat storage. Because fats do not elicit an insulin response, they cannot be stored as body fat.ῶ Insulin takes glucose out of the bloodstream. It is converted first into a starch called glycogen, which is stored in the liver and in muscles. But the body can store only a limited amount of glycogen, so the excess glucose is stored as body fat. This is the process of putting on weight.

When your blood glucose level returns to normal, after about 90 minutes, the insulin level in your bloodstream is still near maximum. As a result, the insulin continues to stack glucose away in the form of fat. Ultimately, the level of glucose in your blood falls below normal, and you feel hungry again. So you have a snack of more carbohydrates, and the whole process starts over again. You're getting fatter, but feeling hungry at the same time. Ultimately, insulin resistance caused by continually high insulin levels in your bloodstream impairs your ability to switch on a satiety center in the brain. You enter a vicious cycle of continuous weight gain combined with hunger. Under such circumstances, it is almost impossible not to overeat. "

I'm not suggesting that we should eliminate all carbs, grains and starches from our diet, but as Dr. Groves explains, our reliance on these foods as the major staples in our diet is hindering our efforts to lose weight and is putting us on a counterproductive weight-gain cycle that counteracts all of our best intentions.

26. Stick to the same daily menu.

A curious habit that I have observed among those who successfully reduce their belly fat and keep their weight under control for long periods of time is the practice of sticking to the same daily menu. I'm not suggesting that they eat the same exact thing every day for breakfast, lunch and dinner (although some do). What I'm suggesting is that they tend to stick to a very limited set of options - all of which incorporates foods they genuinely enjoy.

Getting in the habit of sticking to the same daily menu helps us to predict our daily calorie allotment better because we're not introducing too many "mystery" foods into our diet. It also teaches our taste buds to develop the habit of getting used to foods that are better for us. Additionally, it can also help us to become better attuned to the true calorie and energy needs of our bodies.

When we're constantly eating all kinds of

foods, we're robbing ourselves of the opportunity to introduce healthy routines into our eating patterns. What kinds of healthy foods do you prefer? Maybe it would be a good idea to get into the pattern of consistently eating them instead of allowing your diet to become too varied or experimental.

27. Read food labels.

Even though this was touched on in previous sections, it's probably best that we devote one section just to the concept of reading food labels. Healthy people in our culture are aware of what they're putting in their bodies. Unhealthy people willingly choose to live in blissful ignorance. In the information age that we live in, it's important that we educate ourselves on what we're eating.

Nutrition labels aren't perfect, but they're useful. They make you aware of additives and other strange ingredients and they also help you to understand how many calories you're about to consume. This is important to note.

One of the reasons you may be struggling with excess weight around your mid-section is because, very simply, you're consuming too many calories. The average healthy diet allows for the consumption of approximately 2,000 calories / day, depending on your activity level. If you're eating, drinking and snacking on the wrong foods all day long, you're very likely eating well over 2,000 calories. Some days you may be easily doubling that amount.

It takes a reduction of approximately 3,500 calories to burn a pound of fat or the consumption of an excess 3,500 calories to add a pound of fat. If your caloric intake is too high, it would be a wise and beneficial habit to take a closer look at food labels, not only for the sake of avoiding unhealthy additives and ingredients, but also for the sake of understanding your daily level of calorie consumption.

28. Reward yourself with non-food rewards.

Keeping your motivation level high when you're trying to lose belly fat is critical. As soon as your motivation begins to fade, you will likely find yourself back at square one and that's not something you want to experience, especially after all the effort you've put in to replacing your bad habits with better habits.

Rewarding yourself when you reach personal milestones is a great habit that can promote long-term success, but it's important that you reward yourself in the right way. For most of your adult life, you may have been in the habit of rewarding yourself with food. That's a habit that needs to change. It's a counterproductive habit that can rob you of the fruit of your efforts.

It's better to get in the habit of rewarding yourself with non-food rewards. We all have things that we enjoy that aren't food related. Make a list of some of the things that you like that don't come packed with added calories and give yourself permission to enjoy one of them for each milestone that you reach.

Some ideas that you might want to consider...

>...Treat yourself to a movie if you successfully resisted eating dessert today.

>...Treat yourself to a new pair of pants if your current clothing is becoming too loose.

>...Reward yourself with something that you need for your house (an appliance or a tool) if you've reached one of your major goals.

>...Reward yourself with an afternoon at the spa

Whatever system of rewards you choose, be sure to fill it with a variety of a creative options that will boost your spirits and celebrate your success.   You're doing something that isn't easy and your replacing many long-entrenched habits with better options. Along the way, it's good to reward yourself in ways that will help you reach your next milestone, not push it further away.

29. Don't keep the foods that tempt you in your house.

Have you ever taken a minute to ask yourself, "Which foods tempt me to overeat?" It's a good question to ask because many of these foods are the very things that are contributing to the excess weight around your mid-section.

There are times when your resistance to these foods is going to be low. Maybe you'll have a hard day at work or a disagreement with your spouse. Maybe your kids will damage something that was important to you or irritate you with their disobedience. Maybe you won't even know why you aren't feeling all that great, but because you're not feeling your best, your resistance to tempting snacks is going to be low at times.

If you have these foods within reach, you're very likely to start eating them. If they're just a couple feet away in the pantry, they're going to be in your hand, in your mouth and in your belly before you can count to ten.

A better habit that helps promote the attaining of your long-term goals is to keep those foods OUT OF THE HOUSE. The battle is mostly lost the second they take up room in your cupboard. Your resistance may have been high when you put them away, but a moment of weakness is waiting just around the corner and you're bound to give in to temptation if those tempting snacks are lurking in your kitchen.

Your spouse may protest and your kids may protest, but as much as it depends on you, get in the habit of not bringing your most tempting foods into your home.

30. Take a day off (but just one day).

The final habit on our list is, understandably, the favorite of many people. But a habit that many people who enjoy long-term weight loss enjoy is taking a day off each week from their self-imposed eating restrictions. This may sound counter productive, but evidence seems to indicate that this can help you reach your weight loss goals more effectively than if you never take a day off.

Taking a day to enjoy a little extra food can actually trick your body into working harder to lose weight. Your body is going to look at all of these extra calories and treat them like a foreign invader. It will then kick-start it's defense mechanisms, some of which may have been growing a little lazy or dormant because you've been treating your body so much better. This interruption to the routine can remind your body that you aren't in some sort of starvation mode and your body will in turn continue to work with you to get rid of your excess weight.

Another side benefit of doing this is that it can be a helpful reminder to you of why it's best to continue eating healthy the other six days of the week. Some people notice that at the end of their "cheat day", they feel sluggish and might even experience a mild headache. This helps motive them to get back into the habit of eating better the very next day.

It's important to note that while it may be fun to take a day off from your new eating habits each week, it's very important that one day doesn't become two or three. It can be a slippery slope if you're not careful. One day is fine. Two days is not.

Can I ask for a favor?

I hope you have found this collection of habits to be both helpful and motivational as you seek to shed excess belly fat. Implementing these habits has worked for me and many others and it was my pleasure to put this book together and share them with you.

If you found this book helpful, would you be willing to leave a brief review (even as short as just a couple sentences) on Amazon? Amazon does more to promote books that are reviewed by readers and I would certainly appreciate your help to get this book in the hands of others who could use a word of encouragement. I personally read all reviews that are left by my readers and I'm looking forward to receiving your feedback and hearing your success stories.

I wish you all the best in your efforts! Thanks again!

Sincerely,
Armin Bergmann

Popular Books by Armin Bergmann...

30 Simple Habits for Losing Belly Fat

An easier way to strengthen your body, upgrade your health, improve your appearance and enjoy a better life

30 Simple Habits for Reducing Stress

An easier way to relieve tension, clarify your priorities and enjoy a better life

Drink Yourself Thin

A faster approach to losing weight, gaining energy, detoxing your system and making your skin glow

Drink Yourself Thin - RECIPE GUIDE

The detailed recipe guide for the "Drink Yourself Thin" system

Grain Gut

How cutting just one thing from your diet can rapidly accelerate your weight loss and improve your overall health

Great Abs are Made in the Kitchen

How to lose belly fat by eating the RIGHT foods at the RIGHT time

Walking Off Your Weight With Podcasts

A simple approach to reducing your weight while feeding your mind

Run Faster, Run Smarter

A quick guide for beginners who want to become distance runners

Flat Belly Tips & Tricks

30 simple tips and tricks for getting the flattest belly you've ever had in your life

Diabetic Dieting

The RIGHT way to eat when you're diabetic or looking to transition to a low-carb menu

Printed in Great Britain
by Amazon

12870530R00050